Ten Steps to Fasting

Suzy Dior

ISBN 978-1-387-47341-0

Disclaimer

All this information in the book is for your information only. There is no prescription here; you should ascertain if these are right for you personally. I am not advising you take anything, do anything or advise anyone personally based on this book. This book is for discussion purpose only. Please read this book carefully more than once to obtain the best information and results.

If you are sick you should see a doctor. Nothing written here in this book is to treat any person. You are responsible for your own health. I cannot advise any person in a book because I have never met you. If you feel unwell in any other way you should see a therapist in person.

Introduction

Do you want to lose weight and shrink your waistline quickly? Looking for a miracle cure to help you drop that weight gain, fit into the cute dress …
You can lose five pounds or more per week during this initial phase.
Shedding excess water helps you to feel and look thinner even though the amount of body fat you carry hasn't changed.

The world has changed now and we must look after our own health.

If we don't we could be sick forever as we get left alone. We need to take care of our hearts more and drink lots of water. However if we don't get too fast every year we might find it's too late as we get older. We need to start when we are young to do the fasting regime so that we can find ourselves in a good place as we grow older.

Table of Contents

Step 1

How To Water Fast

The long-term health benefits of water-only fasting are often dependent on dietary and lifestyle modifications. In order to facilitate these changes, I offer educational programs dealing with diet, exercise, proper body use, stress management, sleep, and psychology.

When participants decide to end their fast, they are encouraged to gradually reintroduce food into their diet. This re-feeding process reinforces good dietary habits and typically requires a period of no less than one-half the length of the fast.

For everyday cleansing and healing, occasional 7-10 day fasts combined with regular short fasts such as the one-day (36-hour) water fast should keep you in excellent health.

However, in order to reach the deepest possible level of healing and reap the greatest benefits, it is necessary to dig deeper with a longer fast. For instance, certain serious physical illnesses – those often deemed incurable by Western medicine – require the cleansing of an extended fast in order to permanently heal. Despite what allopathic doctors may tell you, conditions as wide and varied as Type II diabetes, multiple sclerosis, chronic high blood pressure, autoimmune disorders, as well as certain types of tumours are all potentially curable.

I'm privileged to witness this miraculous healing potential of the human body!
You won't starve to death. Unless you're seriously malnourished and underweight to begin with, you carry the better part of 100,000 calories on you, locked in your fat tissue and waiting to be released through ketosis. That's enough to last you well over 40 days. If you're overweight, you could potentially fast for much longer

.

If you continue fasting indefinitely there comes a point where the fast turns into starvation.

Do not fast if you have certain medical conditions. Some medical conditions can be worsened by fasting and can lead to serious health consequences. Do not do a water fast if you have any of the following, unless specifically approved by your doctor:

- Any eating disorder like anorexia or bulimia
- Low blood sugar (hypoglycaemia) or diabetes
- Enzyme deficiency
- Late stage kidney or liver disease[4]
- Alcoholism
- Thyroid dysfunction
- AIDS, tuberculosis, or infectious disease
- Late stage cancer
- Lupus
- Vascular disease or poor circulation
- Heart disease, including heart failure, arrhythmias (especially atrial fibrillation), history of a heart attack, valve problems, or cardiomyopathy
- Alzheimer's disease or organic brain syndrome
- Post-transplant
- Paralysis

Consider starting with a 1-day water fast. Limit your water fast to 3 days if you're doing it on your own. Some evidence suggests that just a 1-3 day short-term fast can have health benefits. If you intend to fast longer than that, only do so under medical supervision – such as at a fasting retreat where you're supervised by a medical professional

Spread out your water consumption throughout the day. Try setting out three one litre jugs every day, so you can see how much water you should drink.

Step 2

Which Sport And Exercise During A Fast?

When you are about to fast you will need to ask yourself which sport you will follow because sport is a big thing in creating weight loss.

You can lose weight easy by stopping dieting, eating, fasting, anything but if you don't do sport as well your body will look thin and wasting away. You do not want that. Do you want a sporting, fit body that looks good to you? I'm going to give you some suggestions and ideas here and you can take some of them and use.. For a start you may need to walk a lot. Then you may need to do some bending and stretching. You may also add some strong Yoga or Chi Gong exercise to it.

Exercise is excellent for reducing your fat. You may like to do it more often. I always do it every morning. You may get up once a day and do your sport. It includes bending, stretching, moving and running.

You can do it like this; walk when you start; and as you get slimmer try to break out into a trot. Nobody is asking you to do a full blown run. Of course if you're used to running you may follow your normal pattern or increase it.

Nobody should get up in the morning and do nothing. Your first pattern is to get up in the morning, move and do some sport. Half an hour is enough. And then do some more later in the day. I suggest one day a week we do nothing but sport. This means your heart rate gets a decent day out once a week. The rest of the week you could do sports once in the morning and once in the afternoon or evening before or after work when you get up or before you go to bed. This includes bending, stretching and increasing your heart rate.

Normally girls do it slower than guys they say but I don't agree. I think girls or ladies can do the same. I don't believe women are limited in any way, as girls or women do sports at excellent rates..

You may like to learn a new sport or do yoga during your fasting period to give you something to think about.

Take your walk from a leisurely stroll to an intense workout by adding intervals. If you aren't a big fan of running or you are just getting back into the swing of cardio or need to give your joints a break...push-ups are one of the most efficient, accessible muscle-building exercises you can do. You can do lots of different variations to make the exercise easier or more difficult according to your weight loss and energy levels

Step 3

How To Do Fruit Juice Fasting

There is one way to fast on fruit juices alone. I used to do it in a retreat centre in Thailand using just watermelon juice for 7 to 10 days. I am a Live blood analyst and used to look at the blood cells of people under the microscope the day before starting the fast and the last day of the fast, to see what condition the blood cells were in before and after fasting. I created the new weight loss program, weighing people before the fast and after the fast to see how much weight loss they had. The results were phenomenal.

Before I came to the retreat, the weight loss program was solely on watermelon juices with herbs, clays and colonics. My opinion after watching thousands of people do the watermelon juice only fast was that there was too much sugar in it.

This was proved in point by the Live blood microscope showing quite clearly that the people who came in without fungi in the bloodstream would leave covered in it. The reason for this is twofold. Firstly, to drink just 5 pints of watermelon juice every day for 10 days with nothing else leaves you internally dehydrated from too much sugar and secondly it's too acidic. The purpose of this retreat was to lose weight.

In order to reduce weight, you need to lose a lot of your sugars. We need to lower our sugars in this society because most people have very high blood sugar. There is only one way to lose sugar and that is to fast it out.

If we just want to lose weight, we may lose it on any diet or fast, as long as we don't exceed our calories. Therefore, a juice fast is for you if you just want to lose weight. To increase that weight loss, you can take a juice that does not have sugars in it or solely a water fast.

When you do a juice fast with fruit you need to make sure the fruit is organic. There is nothing wrong with fruit in the shop as long as it's organic but you must clean it first because little bugs might be on it that can cause havoc with your stomach if you are fasting. This is because you are putting a lot of that fruit into your body and not just one piece.

If you want to fruit juice fast you must do it using freshly squeezed juices. Find yourself a nice big juicer that makes juice easily. I use a Hobbs juicer.. There is no pain like the misery of peeling and cutting forever throughout the days but you have to do it. I liken it to a sword being sharpened, it is too sharp if you catch yourself on it, so be careful please, the same goes for the juicer, do not put your fingers into the machine when it is turned on or you will do yourself an injury. Always use the tool they provide.

After that it's easy. You should be prepared for your fast though so stop and think which week you are going to do your fast. Is it a busy week where you have to go out every day to work? Or can you lay around at home being a fasting individual for the week? Is it on your own? Or will you be doing it with your father or a loved one? The reason is this; you don't want to talk too much about it, just get on with it.

Once you decide your days or week, cancel everything for those days and make sure that there are no surprise dinners or lunches for two.

When you decide to do it, look at all of your calendar except for work, if you have to go there. There are no Massages in this country worth going to because they are so costly but if you go to Thailand you'll find a massage on the beach for £10 in which case you can permanently massage for the rest of your week which is great. If you don't like to do this, have fun in some other way like a herbal bath or decent foot massage to get some of those toxins and fat moving out of your body. That is what it is for. I treat myself daily when on holiday. From fasting to a decent massage or even a facial will do. I liken it to the Ark; there are some small animals but there are some big animals and they are not the same when it comes to every day regular fasting, so be careful with generic advice that's all I will say. If you are a small person, then you may have low blood pressure and will need some extra minerals while you are fasting. Why is that? That is because you have little or no reserves to pull on if you go a bit low on your minerals. So put in a few minerals before you start if you are low blood pressure or a very slim person. I take a tablet called electrolyte deficiency by empirical labs. You can take this if you are underweight but not if you are overweight as it keeps weight on. Doing this keep energy levels up when you are slim and fasting or might keep disease at bay too.

Once you have decided if you are a small person and need to take minerals on your fast because you're not doing it just for weight loss but for purification you need to start eating fresh foods only for a week. This is because the detoxification will be too much for your heart if you don't eat fresh foods beforehand as the toxins would all go to your heart at once. This means no turkey dinners, no huge pieces of cooked meat and no alcohol or drugs. Once you have decided to go cold turkey and not had anything past the usual fresh foods, vegetables, fruits, nuts, seeds, beans and herbs for a week you can then start your fast of juice.

In conclusion a small animal or human should start the detox with fresh food for a few days before the fast to cleanse the system because it will be a huge mass of old junk foods inside if you don't. We need to eliminate during the fast but this can be done by a series of colonics. There is no charge for doing these colonics if you do them indoors by yourself but you may like to have one or two by a practitioner first to see what to do and understand the practice first. Otherwise you will not know how to do it correctly.

You cannot do this on a YouTube or other program it needs to be explained properly by a qualified practitioner. I know, because I used to be one. It is hard to explain the practice online because there are a lot of personal parts, like where does the tube go and what do you do if you pass wind? The reason for the colonic is to empty the bowel completely of old matter. While I completely disapprove of you doing it yourself the first times because it could hurt you, I truly believe all matter should be cleared at least once in the week while you are fasting for the first time.

If you don't take a colonic, then at least try and have an enema.
.
This is one that you buy from the chemist, it's a start, I wouldn't like it for my first retreat but it will empty the lower part of the bowel out if you are stuck. I quite like it on a retreat as well to combine with colonics if you're on a low budget.

When that is over and you have your colonic booked and your enema bought you can then go out and buy the fruit. I suggest a local food shop which can sell you organic food from the shelf or buy a box load because I'm not being rude you're going to get through a lot of fresh fruit. The next thing is buy yourself a juicer if you haven't got one already. There is no right or wrong way to use it just buy the one you like using the best. I have two juicers one is a hand juicer that doesn't use electric so I don't wake anyone up at night! The other one is a posh electric juicer which will whiz round and make a pint of juice in a few minutes.

There is one juicer I prefer to all others and that is the cheap juicer. Why? Because they always end up breaking over time.

Now you have all your tips to get going I suggest you buy your food carefully. What are you going to fast on? Is it going to be apples only? In which case you'll need a lot of apples. Are you going to use a different fruit juice? And why are using that fruit juice? Are you allergic to apples? Or is it because you don't like them.

In Britain we have a lot of apples almost free of charge off the tree or at the shop if you buy in a box load. I would advise a delivery of fresh apple juice if you are busy.

If you're not a small being but you are a big one I would not suggest this fast but I would suggest a fast on vegetables juices only for one week followed by the quick water fast.

Step 4

The Best Way Raw Food Cleansing

The Raw Food Diet is a pure vegetarian diet consisting of mostly raw organic fruits, vegetables, nuts, and seeds. Foods are consumed in their natural whole state and not heated above 118° F.

As we all know, the foundation of a healthy raw food diet is raw fruits and vegetables. But, most of these vegetables lose their vitamins, minerals and enzymes when they are cooked.

A raw food diet is based on unprocessed and uncooked plant foods like fresh fruit and vegetables, sprouts, seeds, nuts, grains, beans, nuts, dried fruit, and seaweed. A strict follower will avoid all meat, fish, fowl and dairy. The idea is to consume food that is as natural and unprocessed as possible.

There are many chefs around the world who have come out with their own versions of raw food recipes but the main concept is to make the recipe from raw uncooked vegetables and fruits.

Here we will be discussing a few things which make perfect ingredients for raw food recipes:

Green smoothies: Take a cup of water, add a cup of frozen or fresh blueberries, 2-3 ripe bananas and blend them all in a blender. You will feel rejuvenated, the diet is really filling and you will consume lot more nutrients compared to your normal breakfast.

Blended Salad: A blended salad can do wonders both to your stomach as well as digestive system. We all know the benefits of salads and that is why we consume salads every day in bits and pieces. When you are on a raw food diet, it is recommended to take a whole plate full of salads anytime of the day. You can have the following ingredients:

2-3 medium tomatoes, roughly chopped
4 leaves lettuce (big)
1 big handful spinach
1 green onion

1 cucumber.

All these things make a perfect salad which you can take anytime of the day.

Bananas – Bananas are a perfect add on to Raw food recipes. You can take them anytime of the day either in a solid state or just mix them with water, blueberries and make a shake. They not only make you feel full but also helps in digestion.

Coconut water – Coconut water acts as a great appetiser. It not only makes a perfect add on with raw foods but also helps in keeping the body temperature to the optimum level.

Mango – Mangoes are also great to include in raw food recipes. You can use various combination of mangoes with blueberry, raspberry and make a shake for yourself.

Apart from these there are various other things which you can add to make some amazing raw food recipes but these are main ingredients one should have. Raw food recipes have really helped people adopt a healthy lifestyle and it doesn't cost a fortune to actually make raw food recipes.

Raw food diet has been the centrepiece of the eyes since last few years. The concept has actually been applied more and more by people since its advantages are numerous. It doesn't involve starving yourself in order to lose those extra toxins from your body. Not only toxins, but people who have switched to raw food diet have actually felt better both physically and mentally. Raw food diet will also give you a reduction in weight.

The raw food diet is actually a concept wherein you are dependent on raw fruits, vegetables and juices for your daily needs. You completely switch off from the unhealthy, cooked food which usually takes away all the necessary nutrients.

Usually a Raw food diet is undertaken by people for a period of 7-14 days but people who have successfully completed this phase have actually found out that raw food diet is actually the best thing to have and have switched to it partially if not completely.

Components of Raw food diet:

- A raw food diet normally includes lots of fruits, green vegetables and drinking lots of water.

A transition menu needs to be especially flexible, as often cravings for junk foods and sweet foods, as well as other addictive substances can appear out of the blue and put a very real spanner in the works. By ensuring that you fully satisfy your hunger at every meal with fresh fruits, salads and organic whole foods, you will actually start feeling good from inside as the toxins from the body are washed away. You will feel more active, your skin looks fresh and better.

Breakfast: A typical raw food breakfast can include a glass full of fresh fruit juice or a whole bowl of fresh fruits. Fruits have enzymes which react with the body and cut out toxins and excess waste from your body. If you are really hungry, you can have a plate of fresh fruit salad or vegetable salad after a couple of hours. A glass of lemon water also does wonders as it greatly helps in removing the toxins and waste from your body.

Lunch: You can actually have a green vegetable soup which can also include tomatoes, sprouts, cucumbers. Include lemon juice as an add on.

Dinner: You can finish the day with a big filling salad. Some of the toppings you can use are nuts and seeds, olives, tomatoes, sprouts, chopped cucumber and carrot. Remember the point here is not to starve yourself but to actually convert to a healthy lifestyle and your diet plays a major role in contributing to a healthy lifestyle.

Raw Food Cleanse

Raw Food cleanse or raw food detox diet is a concept which has been discovered a few years back and has helped many people lose both weight and harmful toxins from their body. Raw food cleanse is basically a concept wherein the person depends completely on uncooked raw food for his/her daily nutrition and just eats raw uncooked food.

The reason why raw foods are getting popular is because of the fact that our body really starts to react to the starch, sugar and added preservatives present in the food and we quickly start to gain weight as well as have other harmful effects on the health. Raw foods act as a routine breaker and help rejuvenate both mind and body as you will be completely off the junk food and will take only good nutritious food which will flush out all the toxins from your body.
Raw food is just what you think it would be: any food that has been uncooked, untreated, or unadulterated.

No matter where you stand on raw food, everyone agrees that consuming more fresh greens, vegetables, fruits, fats, and proteins is an excellent way to reach or maintain your optimal health.

Apples, apricots, raisins, grapefruit, bananas, pineapple, blackberries, blueberries, cantaloupes, cherries, dates, figs, grapes, honeydew melon, kiwi, lemons, limes, mangos, nectarines, oranges, papaya, peaches, pears, persimmons, plums, pomegranates, raspberries, strawberries, and watermelon are a few most popular raw fruits which most of the people take and we also suggest you the same because they simply work for the body.

Usually people stick to juices, uncooked vegetables and fruits when on a detox. The process starts usually with getting off the cooked meal completely and being more dependent on raw fruits and vegetables. Cooked food has a tendency to lose all the nutrients and what you actually eat is just food which tastes good but without having any nutrition in particular.

Often, this raw food cleanse is undertaken for a period of 7 days to 14 days and if done properly, the body can lose a lot of toxins and excess body weight. We have seen those movie actors and actress. They indulge in frequent detox to remove unwanted fats as well as look amazing.

The best part about this raw food cleanse is that you do not have to stress nor starve yourself. It is basically eating food which is not cooked.
There are a few people who might experience symptoms like vomiting and nausea in the first few days. This is common and is the effect of not eating the daily food that you habitually eat.

Once you realise the benefits of raw food and juices you will actually want to avoid cooked food and will be hooked to the raw food.

Gourmet Raw Food Recipes!

Raw food is almost always healthier than the foods that most of us are choosing every day. If you eat only fresh, unprocessed foods, you will automatically cut out all refined sugars and flours and most fatty foods. During a raw cleanse, you will eat very simply and your body will thank you for that!

The raw food cleanse can last from 7 to 10 days. You will need to do some planning ahead of time.

Social occasions can be difficult when you are eating raw so if you want to make your detox as easy as possible, try to pick a period of time when you do not have any business lunches, restaurant meals or visits to family.

If people are visiting, you that's fine because you can control what you eat. It is possible to take your own food when eating at somebody else's house but it can be hard for them to understand so it will be much simpler if you can find a clear week in your diary for a cleanse.

The day before your raw food cleanse begins, try to eat as simply as possible with plenty of fruit and vegetables. Avoid eating a lot of meat or fatty, sugary foods and stay off alcohol.
If you drink more than two cups of coffee/tea per day, cut down gradually in the days leading up to the cleanse to avoid caffeine withdrawal headaches during the cleanse.

Then begin your raw food cleanse with a 24 hour fast, starting from the time that you finish your evening meal on the last day before the cleanse. So imagine I am starting a cleanse on a Saturday.

I eat dinner on Friday evening, finishing at 7.30 pm. I don't eat or drink anything else after that except water, until 7.30 pm on Saturday, day 1 of the cleanse. Then I will have my first raw food meal.

During the raw food cleanse you will eat anything that is the fresh, non-fatty fruit, leaves, stem or roots of a plant, without cooking it. This includes salad, vegetables and fruits. You can have as much of these as you like, whenever you like, but do be sure to include at least one pound of green vegetables every day. This will give you a broader range of minerals than if you eat fruit only, which means you will have fewer cravings. Celery is great if you have cravings for salty foods.

Be sure to have a wide variety of ripe fruits and vegetables in the house at all times during your raw food cleanse. It is important to be able to have whatever type of fruit or vegetable you feel like eating.

Foods to Avoid on a raw food cleanse.

There are a few fatty fruits that you should avoid. These include avocado, coconut and durian (jackfruit). You will also avoid nuts, seeds and oils. There is no need for any dried herbs or seasonings, although you can use fresh herbs in small quantities if you want.

You will not need any drinks other than water. Be sure to wash all foods well.

You can make a simple salad dressing by blending equal quantities of tomato and cucumber in the blender. Add a few herbs or red bell pepper if you want.

If you want to continue eating a raw food diet after the end of the cleanse, you can add some fats in the form of nuts, avocado, unpasteurised cheese etc. The cleanse program does not contain all of the fatty acids and other nutrients that are needed for a long term diet.

Be aware that you may have some detox symptoms in the first few days of the cleanse and in some cases these can be quite severe. Check with your medical adviser before going on a raw food cleanse, especially if you are pregnant or nursing or have any pre-existing medical conditions.

If you do not raw food fast, then you should go on a detoxification fast instead to clear your toxins from your mind, body and soul. This will make you lose your addictions to biscuits, fast foods, alcohol, drugs and medications. If you are with the doctor check with them first to make sure these rules apply to you. I cannot be responsible for medications as they are not my line of work you should go to your doctor for this. If you should see your doctor, make sure it's a good one who knows your goals and dreams and can follow you through to the end. I in no way condemn these medications but if you should have nuts and seeds allergies just see an allergist or a specialist in therapy of some kind of your choosing. Leave out what doesn't suit your stomach, or any other part of you or any foods that you do not like either.

Have fun, have a great week.

Step 5

How To Fast In Moderation?

Health Benefits of Fasting One Day a Week

From an alimentary point of view, fasting means not eating and not drinking anything at all. Not eating anything and drinking just water is also considered fasting.

However, some experts question this statement, as they claim that fasting in a proper way means that one shouldn't eat or drink anything.
When the body is deprived of food, there will be systemic cleaning, except for vital tissues.

Fasting is also an important part of many religions, and some experts believe that fasting can do wonders for people's health.

How Does It Work?

From a technical standpoint, the body reacts to fasting after the first 24 hours, but chemically, food shortages determine the use of carbohydrate reserves as an energy source.
The liver is responsible for converting fat into a chemical substance called ketone (the substance that results from the metabolism of acetic acid and beta-hydroxybutyric acid), and then it distributes these organisms throughout the body via the bloodstream.

When fat is used this way, free fatty acids are released into the bloodstream and are used by the liver as an energy source. The more a person eats less, the more the body pushes these fatty deposits and creates more ketones (accumulation referred to in ketosis' case).

The starvation issue only arises when the body will be forced to use vital tissue to survive.

Fear related to muscle fibres decrease due to protein catabolism is unjustified. Even after a long fast, the number of muscle fibres remains the same. Although the size and strength of healthy cells can be reduced, they are not affected.

Fasting is an alimentary therapeutic method practiced in specialised clinics in several countries around the world. There are many renowned clinics in Austria, Germany, Switzerland, France, Britain, Russia, the USA, Japan, and China.

Step 6

How To Do A Vegetable Juice Fast

Juice FASTING

A person doing a juice FAST consumes only the juices from fresh fruits and vegetables, in as many times a day as they like and can comfortably drink, in place of their solid food meals.

The amount of juices drunk a day is 2-3 litres/quarts a day. In between juices, you may also drink vegetable soups, herbal teas, and plenty of pure drinking water. In other words, it is a purely liquid, nutritious diet.

With this kind of juice fast, healing reactions may occur earlier in the fast and possibly more severe, but consider them all as good signs of your body being on the way to healing!

Juice FEASTING

- There are various interpretations of juice feasting, though for me, juice FEASTING means consuming juiced (1-2 litres/quarts a day) and EATING fresh fruits and vegetables.

- You may include lightly cooked vegetables (steamed, lightly stir-fried, or blanched), during your juice feasting. The idea is not to be hungry, and you can eat as much as you comfortably want, without forcing yourself.

- During juice feasting, you eliminate all other harmful foods from your diet: Flour and sugar products, processed and deep-fried foods, dairy and meat products, soda, alcohol and caffeine.

SHOULD YOU JUICE FAST OR JUICE FEAST?

YOU decide whether you want to juice fast or juice feast. There are no hard and fast rules.

Some people like to keep it simple by drinking only juices, along with water, broths, and herbal teas. This is great, it works!

Some people cannot afford to go hungry so prefer to eat alongside juicing. They go on a juice FEAST as described above. Feasting on fresh, organic food is the key in healing. This works too.

Whatever you decide to do, it is a detox/juice cleanse that's unique for you. Drinking an increased amount of juices provides you a variety of nutrients which you would otherwise not get.

The amount you drink determines how fast you will heal from your ailment. YOU decide how fast you want your healing.

Juice feasting is suitable for you, if you are diabetic or suffer from hypo/hyperglycaemia, but stick with green juices only.

If you will be or have just undergone a surgery, a juice feast may be the perfect diet for your situation, although scaled down in quantity. There is one way to scale it down if you're lost and don't know what to decide:
If you're not losing weight on your fasting option, then you are not doing it properly.

It is about FASTING not putting excessive amounts of any foods or juice in your body!
You want to be weight conscious unless you are underweight, in which case this will not apply to you. But still be careful of your sugar loading on sweet juices and fruits.

There is nothing to learn, just avoid sweet juices unless you are consciously on a sweet juice fast in which case beware you don't PUT ON weight!
The best juices are vegetable juices in small doses.

YOUR COMPLETE GUIDE TO A SUCCESSFUL JUICE FAST

You will naturally have many more questions about juice fasting which are answered in my book.

If you are seriously considering a juice fast/feast, please thoroughly read up all you can about it. Come with me as I share with you from my personal experience.

Before we go further, there are two very important factors we need to consider:

The current state of your health
You MUST NOT attempt a juice fast if your current state of health falls under any of these categories mentioned below:

- You're pregnant or nursing.
- You have any kind of eating disorders (then close supervision is vital for the success of your healing).
- You are on daily prescription medication. Please consult with a health professional who is skilled in nutrition or detoxification. You MUST NOT discontinue or reduce your medication on your own accord.
- If you have a kidney or liver disease, you're anaemic, have low blood pressure, a terminal disease, epilepsy or any other chronic conditions, it is not advisable to juice fast/feast UNLESS you're on Gerson Therapy. (This topic is currently not covered on this site.)

Juice fasting/feasting is best for individuals who have health problems and WANT to get well. If you fall under the above categories, you should fast only under close supervision of a health professional.

If/when you decide to go on a juice fast/feast, do get acquainted with all the implications, and know what to expect in order to benefit most from your juice fast. You don't want unwelcome surprises.

Is your juicer safe to use for juice fasting?

All that I have to say here about doing a safe juice fast includes using a safe juice extractor. I often discourage use of a centrifugal juicer for a juice fast as it may do more harm to you than good. Please read about whether your juicer is safe.

If you can, invest in a slow juicer that will last you a lifetime in providing you fresh juices in the best form.
Another disadvantage of using a centrifugal juicer is that it's not as effective for juicing green vegetables which are the most important ingredients in a healing fast.

Also, a word of caution, by using a centrifugal juicer, the result of your juice fast may not be as optimum as if you would use a gear juicer.

I've had people tell me that they get well too using a centrifugal juicer. Fine with that. But I've also come across people whose health had deteriorated even though drinking juices over the years, which I discovered were extracted using centrifugal juicers.

The cause may or may not be the type of juicer used, but, understanding what oxidation does to the body, I would not take the chances of drinking oxidized juices. You decide which way you want to go.

WHEN IS THE BEST TIME OF THE YEAR TO JUICE FAST/FEAST?

There is no doubt that juice fasting is a great thing to do to detoxify and to heal a health condition. However, when it comes to deciding on the time of the year to juice fast, there are a few things you need to consider.

First of all, consider where you live. If you live in a place that is hot and humid all-year round, such as countries near the Equator, then juice fasting at any time of the year is an easy decision. Any time is a good time!

But, if you live in colder countries where there are four seasons, such as in the northern or southern hemispheres, then it might be helpful to juice fast during the warmer months.

Here's why …

Freshly-extracted juices are generally more "cooling" in nature. For example, during winter, your body will tend to crave a bowl of hot soup, rather than to drink a glass of watermelon juice.

Well, occasionally you may want to drink a watermelon juice on a cold day, but your body will certainly not take well to drinking fresh "cooling" juices every day for weeks on end.

During cold months, your body needs to eat solid, hot, cooked food to keep warm. But if you juice fast during the winter, it may lower your body temperature further, thus may cause an uncomfortable feeling of being constantly cold.

If you simply have to juice fast during the winter for whatever your reasons, there are ways to work around it:

Do juice FEASTING to include lightly-cooked food in your regime.

Include as many of these body-warming foods as you can in your juices and meals.

- Add spices in your juices and foods.
- Drink hot broths and soups.
- Drink herbal teas.
- The idea is to be creative, to make it work for you.

HOW TO JUICE FAST: EVERYTHING YOU NEED TO KNOW

There are many things you should know before you start a juice fast, especially if you're new to juicing. In this complete guide to juice fasting, I cover everything you need to know before you start a juice fast. Some of these topics, you may not even have thought about.

1. Juice fasting benefits:
People juice fast for various reasons. Some juice fast to detoxify—to "reset the internal button", some juice fast for healing, others juice fast to lose weight.
For whatever reason you're fasting, two very important benefits take place when you juice fast—you allow your digestive system to rest, and for your body to heal.

2. Why you need to juice fast:
If you experience any side-effects such as headache or tiredness this is partly due to the toxins your expelling from your system due to the fast. This will pass and you will feel much better later.

3. How to prepare for your juice fast:
Doing a juice fast requires some work—shopping for your fruits and vegetables, cutting them up, juicing and washing.

4. Stages of juice fasting:
You think you've decided on the number of days to juice fast.
Everybody is at their different stages of their lives and health. But, when you go on a juice fast journey, you will begin to feel changes in your body, depending on how long you juice fast. Be equipped with this information so you know what to expect and do not experience some unwanted surprises.

5. Keeping a journal on your juice fast journey:
Do not leave everything to memory. Most of the time, we cannot even recall what we ate for lunch two days ago. There are many benefits to keeping a juice fast journal to help you keep track of what worked and what didn't.

6. What to expect on a juice fast:
Whether you are on a short juice fast or on an extended juice fast, you are bound to experience some symptoms that you don't normally experience.

There may be some more intense aches and pains, nausea or bloating. When you expect them, it will be easier when you actually experience them. These are all positive signs that something is working inside your body towards healing.

7. Healing reactions during a juice fast:
Should you decide to go on an extended juice fast for therapeutic purposes, you may experience some physical healing reactions, or sometimes called "healing crisis".
With extended juice fasts, you may also experience emotional healing reactions. The emotional reactions may not be pleasant and sometimes even seem scary, but they are necessary as you walk through the healing process, and purge them out of your system.
Suppressed negative emotions and trauma get stored in your deep tissues as toxins. And with deep cleansing through extended juice fasts, they can be expelled, bringing much-needed relief.

8. How much juice to drink on a juice fast:
When you juice fast, you have to make a conscious effort to drink enough fluid throughout the day. The key to juice fasting is hydration with all the natural vitamins, minerals and enzymes. So what helps with hydration, and how much is enough?

9. How to store freshly-pressed juices for longer:
This is a common question most people ask when they start juicing. If you're going on a juice fast, chances are you will want to make more juices and store them so you don't spend time juicing and washing all the time!
I discuss some tips on how to have your freshly-pressed juices keep for longer. Storage options also play an important part in ensuring that your juices stay as fresh as possible.

10. Juice fast plans:
So you've come this far and decided to go on a juice fast. I have prepared a few juice fast plans, divided into one week, two weeks, three weeks and beyond. Each article will discuss how you can prepare for the program, what you can expect during and after the juice fast.

11. Juice fast recipes:
If you're new to juice fasting, you may be curious about what to include in your juicing. You can use almost any fruits and vegetables. If you have a blood sugar issue, then stick with more green vegetable juices; green apples and lemons are permitted.

As for me, there are a few fruits and vegetables that I usually use when doing a juice fast. I make them all in large quantities and store in my fridge for up to 3-4 days.

Learn about these ingredients that you can also use for your juice fast recipes and the reasons why you should use them. You can get creative and mix and match them.

12. Juice fast tips for working people:

With a little planning, juice fasting can work well for you even if are out at work most part of the day and the week.

We discuss some practical tips that you can use to make juice fasting work for even busy people like you.

13. Supplements when juice fasting – do you need them?

This is valid question commonly asked by those going on a juice fast: "What about fibre, protein and supplements when juice fasting?"

Learn what fruits and vegetables that can provide you protein, and most of all the nutrients that your body needs during the juice fast, for detoxing and nourishing.

14. Writing your own shopping list:

By now, you should have an idea on how long you want to go on your juice fast. A little planning helps you to reduce wastage.

There is no "one list fits all". Every individual has different needs, different budget, different type of juicers (means you get different juice yield) and different purposes. Here are some things to consider.

15. Lymphatic massage to supercharge your juice cleanse:

Doing a juice fast is a great way to detoxify and flush your body of harmful toxins to revitalise our entire body. When you combine your juice fast with some massage, it can help increase the effectiveness of the detox.

There are self-massage methods that you can do to get your lymph fluid moving properly to promote easier detoxification.

16. How to break a juice fast safely:

Breaking fast is an important part of your entire juice fast journey. Breaking fast safely and responsibly will ensure the end-results of your juice fast go a long way.

I give you some advice here on how you can break your fast gently and safely, with suggestions on some foods that you can eat, and when you can introduce them back into your diet.

17. Juice fasting for weight loss:

The main reason for doing a juice fast is usually for health reason. A juice fast detoxifies your body of toxins, then nourish it back to health.

When you go on a juice fast, you may initially see a big weight loss—this is your body water weight loss. After that the weight loss may plateau. Your body is intelligent in that it knows what to fix first in your body, and weight loss will follow.

An extended juice fast including mostly green vegetable juices would be more effective for weight loss.

Step 7

How To Do A Five-Day Fasting Retreat

Can't Get to a Health Retreat This Year? Here's How to Create a Five-Day Health Programme.

In the current climate attending a health retreat is clearly off the agenda, but it doesn't mean you can't get the benefits of rejuvenating mini break in the comfort of your own home.

I've teamed up with some experts and created some simple tips to be used in conjunction with a five-day fasting detox, to help you create an at-home health reset and an environment for your emotional wellness to thrive.

Get prepared:
One of the main reasons people fail to follow through with any healthy routine is a lack of preparation. The old adage of 'by failing to prepare you are preparing to fail' applies here. Set yourself a routine. Plan to spend some time offline and include a digital detox element to your wellbeing retreat and remove the temptation of lockdown baking snaps on social media. Remove tempting snacks or trigger foods from your home. This way, you don't have to summon willpower every time you open the cupboard or make the mistake of having a big gorge the day before your fast starts.

Nutrition:
A five-day fast mimicking diet could be the perfect way to give your body the break it needs to detox, regenerate and restore vital energy. Combined with mindful practises, yoga, meditation and spa rituals, this at home reset could be the perfect way to reset and get ready for re-entry to the outside world.
Leading health retreats often use fasting as a scientifically backed way to detox the body and improve mental clarity but fasting without supervision is challenging and potentially dangerous.

Mindfulness:
Many people report mental focus and clarity during the five-day fast mimicking diet. This is the perfect time to download a mindfulness app and get into a good meditation practice. If you download the Calm app there are plenty of five-day programmes to tackle various issues from sleep to anxiety, so why not time one of these to align with your five-day at-home retreat?

Exercise:
Light exercise is recommended with a focus on restorative activities like yoga and walks, ideally in nature. The fast is designed for rest and rejuvenation, so vigorous exercise is not recommended. During the first couple of days of the fast, the body uses up circulating blood sugar and stored glycogen (glucose stored in muscles and liver cells) and burns more stored body fat for energy. From day three autophagy is unregulated. Autophagy is a process that helps maintain healthy cellular function, encouraging cells to repair and regenerate. The least number of calories are consumed on days three and five, so on those days take time to go for gentle walks and explore your area by foot. On the other days try yoga to flex and stretch your body. There are plenty of stretching and yoga apps and YouTube videos available to help enhance your regime. Try the free '30 Day Splits' app which has a simple, 20-minute routine to help improve flexibility with a series of stretches.

Sleep:
In individuals with balanced blood sugar levels, intermittent fasting has been shown to support improved sleep quality, so work on further enhancing your bedtime regime and promoting healthy sleep behaviours. Turn your phone off at least an hour before bedtime and have a relaxing bath with magnesium salts before bed to help you unwind. Having a regular sleep and wake time can also help to promote a stable body clock and improved sleep.

Baths:
On the subject of bathing, a bath is a wonderful calming "me time" ritual to give yourself 20 minutes in the bath and a little time to relax and gather yourself afterwards. To help you float away, try breathing in through the nose for five seconds and out through the mouth for five seconds, increasing to ten seconds for each, and continuing for two minutes. Soaking by candlelight will give you a spa-like experience! Dimming the lights and lighting a candle will also help with the relaxation process.

So, what can you expect when you complete your five-day fast? In a published human trial, one 5-day fast resulted in an average of 5 pounds of weight loss and a 1-inch loss of fat around the waistline. Not only is it a quick and efficient way to lose weight, a five-day fast will also stimulate cellular rejuvenation, support metabolic health and promote healthy ageing. Not to mention renewed energy and a sense of calm from your at-home spa experience!

Step 8

Why Attend a Fasting Retreat Abroad?

Fasting in Europe: Detox in Comfort!

Kick start your diet with a cleansing fast in Europe. With a fresh digestive system, detoxed organs and an improved immune system, you'll find reaching and maintaining a healthy weight much easier.

During a fast your calorie intake is reduced dramatically and sometimes food is omitted altogether. A large amount of water and special fasting teas are recommended throughout the fast to keep you hydrated and energised and to flush out toxins. Guests on a fasting holiday, report finding it much easier than doing a fast alone. You are with like-minded people facing the same challenges, round the clock therapy and spa-treatments and an experienced fasting specialist who designs your personalised diet and programme. There couldn't be a more relaxing way to fast!

Why attend a fasting retreat abroad?

Schroth, Buchinger and F.X Mayr where the fasting methods were all developed, is widely considered to be the homeland of fasting and detox retreats. The stunning landscapes of Hungary and Slovenia also offer an idyllic backdrop for your fasting holiday in Europe, or those desiring a warmer climate can undertake fasting programmes in sunny Portugal.

In an abroad retreat fasting includes some of the following usually:

- Mind blowing views.
- Lovely long walks in scenic nature.
- Some of the World's Best fasting teachers and their students who are far accomplished in the world.
- Often some yoga teacher extraordinaire who has come a long way to see you and therefore offers a good structure with mantras.

33

- Gurus of many nationalities may show up at your retreat and you might enjoy their good and cheering company
- Often Sports people and their own gurus are there!
- Other attractions are:
- Clean and healthy younger therapists who know their stuff
- Walks along miles of grand canals.
- Tours of history.
- Lovely old museums.
- Friends that are new to you.

Step 9

Mind, Body and Spirit in Fasting

There is nothing past price and holiday time that will set you apart from a home retreat.

Although holidays are a past thing in the pandemic I am sure that will pass.

You can try and do your own retreat indoors. It's cheaper, easier and useful to do on your own because of pandemic, social situations or your own reasons. I like fasting indoors as it's relaxing and cheaper. There is nothing to lose either, just a few cakes down the drain before you start as I don't keep fruits or cakes indoors when I am fasting due to temptation. That applies to all foods really! I don't clear out the cupboards properly but any junk foods I take out of the house before I start. That is because when you finish fasting you don't really feel like junk foods any more. Obviously it also stops you cheating on your fasting retreat at home.

If you should attend a fasting retreat abroad then look for the one that is easiest or quickest to get to as it makes all the difference. There is a huge cost difference in the nearest country to yours vs a huge Thai holiday which will cost you a fortune. The secret is to save money while going there so you can achieve another abroad holiday soon after to show off your tan! There's nothing quite like having a 'beach babe' body plus a nice tan on holiday to keep you going. And that is what is keeping you going during your fast is to keep reminding yourself you are going on holiday to show it off after. There is nothing quite like five pounds of body fat off you or more to keep you going faster on your fast.

It's a nice feeling also, lighter, tanned and feeling good from all the sunlight and massages you'll find abroad. Also, there will be like minded friends on your retreat abroad to keep you going and soak up the sunlight with you. You might like it better than staying at home but the option is yours.

It's good to say some positive affirmations daily like:

My body is healthy; my body is slim!
Or
My clothes fit me easily and I enjoy looking good.
Or
I feel healthier and fitter every day!

You might try some new visualizations which take your nearer to the top as well!!

Mine are to imagine an older self. A self, past the sell by date as they say!! And see her looking as great as I am today, positive, younger, slimmer and more vibrant. Saying, this is what I want to look like as I get old. Then visualizing the older you on a good day, say to her, what do you want I should do in order to be like you at that age?
And hear her reply.

To do this you need to be laid flat on your couch, counselling yourself quietly. You may like to take someone else along on this for the ride but be careful that someone else doesn't hold you back from your true self. Plant the seed carefully that they too will be at their utmost positive self for you and for themselves too.

Visualize yourself like this, every single day and you will be positively your best when you grow older.

Look back at your younger self today from that space of being an older woman and say to the younger you, what you need to hear from her, to be the best version of yourself today? Do what you need to do in order to survive a very long time. Keep your hair in good condition, your feet in great show condition and look after your teeth for a very long time to come they will serve you. You cannot get by in life without all parts of your body working optimally for you. Keep a plan to reduce weight if you need to and work with it to eliminate any toxins from the heart up. Then you can be well for life.

There is another visualization you can do from the alternate angle and this is what you do…

1.Lie flat on your back prepare to visualize.

2.Ask yourself what an older you would look like if she is at her worst?

3. Then from that place ask the older woman who is at her worst what would she advise you to do in life right now to avoid that worst place and let her reply.

4. Sometimes you will get a worthwhile goal, treat or angle on perspective that will let you survive for a bit longer. Do not start to worry that this is what you'll end up like! As we all aim to goal set most years and most likely you'll over ride it.

Pretty you.
What goals could you set to extend your horizons to a prettier you?
Ask yourself what would you like to do in your future that you've not done yet?
Think about lives that you have not lived yet and wonder if you can do it too?

Like writing books in the Pandemic was something I had wanted to do for a long time but I had put it off saying I was too busy or too past it!

Could you too do a goal that causes you to pause?

- Like climbing the Himalayas?
- Creating a new farm yard school to give young animal lessons?
- Or using your well-being to create another farm scene that schools young people to lose inhibitions and just be themselves?

There are so many things you could manage just in your own town if you could put it into words. Take a few moments to write it all down.

There is NOTHING which will stop you if you put your mind to it during this fasting time. Everything comes into perspective during fasting to give you a new momentum when you do a 7 day non-stop fast.

- You might fall in love?
- Get a new dog?
- Find a new way to work?

Use the time wisely to shore up your life and find new ways of working with others to give you your dream life ahead.

Have fun with it:

- Do it in nature
- Do it with a friend.

- Tell each other what your dreams are?
- Give her support and work out what to do together?
- Do her dreams too and find new ways to work together which will give you both soul and meaning.
- We are not meant to work together but working in a team will both inspire you and help you to understand new things.
- Give your new ideas a dream board and cut out pretty pictures to put on your wall for the future, reminding you new ideas are about to spring forth!

Step 10

After The Fast

Following your fasting period however long or short and whatever type of fasting you have decided to do will help you get thin. Then you may break the fast and continue on your new lifestyle at home.

On the last day of your fast prepare to break it by looking at your soup mixer and not your juicer for a change. Buy a blender otherwise if you don't have a soup mixer.

Options for breaking the fast are shown below quite clearly. Don't fall into the trap of breaking it with alcohol and clearly not junk food or heavy foods from the cooker immediately, although a light steamed meal will be fine.

Option 1:

Juice daily from now on and add foods as required.
First start with raw vegetables on the dish mixed and grated lightly for an easy digestion the first and second days.
Third day you may add a fruit dish on top of the mixed vegetables and lightly stir fried vegetables in small amounts.
Fourth day add some of your favourite protein, maybe meat, fish, eggs or seeds daily from now on.
Fifth day add some sugars like dates, pineapples, surprise yourself with homemade chocolates or parcel together a wrap for yourself. See if you can do it yourself at home because it's cheaper and lighter on the heart and the stomach to do this for yourself.
Sixth and seventh days do what you feel like doing but keep it light as you don't want to put back on the pounds again!

If you don't know by now, you should be exercising once a week or twice daily depending on what your current schedule is like. Don't overdo it but neither should you under do it. 3000 calories need to be burnt off daily.

Keep your fasting regime under your belt and use it for when you put on the extra pounds again.

Option 2.

Have a day on, day off juice fast once you are finished to keep it going a while longer, lose some more weight or just to stay healthy and fit.
You can lose weight for longer this way and avoid looking skinny too as you weight on and weight off daily!

Just start with one fruit juice a day and top up with exercise from a bike or daily swimming on top to lose the most weight and tone up those fat muscles. Exercise is fitness but it's also muscle toning on top and if we want to look fit and healthy it's important to tone those muscles for good. Just cycling won't do it, you need one other form of exercise too. Well done if you're doing it already.

The second day where you eat will be yours to do with what you like but eat sensibly instead of your daily binging which got you into the overweight situation in the first place.

First of all, diet has got to be safe. So, don't overload on carbs and biscuits, instead bring into your life a few decent proteins and put back in minerals from organic vegetables at farms near you.

The proteins have to be decent in that they are free range. Incorporate it into your lifestyle and you will be young and healthy for a long time. Become vegetarian and put in beans, mushrooms, lettuce, legumes and everything you see in the gardens around you and on the shelves, except one thing – rapeseed oils. Don't be aware too much but eat decent oils such as olive oil if you must put extra oil on things or butter and coconut oil for simple sterol fats.

That means you cook for yourself, as supermarkets and other stores put mercenary liquids into their fried and cooked foods such as rapeseed and other oils which simply shouldn't be in the body today.

Take care not to overcook your foods. They become soggy and unlike natural foods you used to eat. Try buying a steamer or using your mother's old recipes.

No fast foods..

Fried foods are out.

Try steaming dishes.

You should be good for life..!

Write down here some of your goals: